777 wrote: I found this a wonderful, concise description of muscle testing

I found this a wonderful, concise description of muscle testing that I can recommend to friends. This is a quick read with information on effective use of muscle testing AKA energy testing or "applied kinesiology." It does not drag or bog down, just describing how it works, how to do it, and how to keep from doing it wrong.

I greatly appreciate this handout length "book" so I can point other people to it when I would like something to help validate any introduction of the topic to friends and acquaintances. I also appreciate that there is nothing too vague or ethereal in the brief explanation, describing that muscle testing works by the electrical energy flowing or not flowing in a muscle. I was very interested to learn some new ways and viewpoints on inhibitions to successful muscle testing outcomes.

I also enjoyed learning about the author's story and background with EFT.

Helen83 wrote: This book really helped me
So much more than muscle testing! If you're interested in changing your life, reading this is a great choice. Valuable resource!

Tom Brodie wrote: Finally!
While my story doesn't involve gas lines, I had a similar experience that drove me to work with both western and alternative practitioners. I also did an internship with an energy

healer; anyway, I've been trying to learn how to do this for years, but I've had two wrist surgeries and a dull sense of touch in one hand.

This little book is great! It provided several techniques that work for me.

Long time customer wrote: Well written and informative
Excellent job!!! I've used muscle testing on and off for years without understanding what was happening, and not happening at times. Tessa gives clear, simple instructions with a variety of different ways to test; with another person or by oneself. I didn't realize there were so many ways to check even whether a supplement would be beneficial for my health. I highly recommend this book and author.

John C. wrote: 5 Star Self Help
I like what I learned in this book. It was very informative. I knew about and used muscle testing myself, even so I learned a good amount I didn't know. I recommend this book for anyone interested in the topic it covers.

Thomas Pranio wrote: Excellent Book!
Okay, this subject matter might be a little esoteric but the way it is presented is not. Well written, fun to experiment with the drills and experiences presented.

Jacqueline wrote: Learn to muscle test on yourself properly.
I discovered just the right technique for me. And I was able to overcome some obstacles that were causing me to get mixed results. This book is excellent for people who want to muscle test on themselves.

Linda wrote: Very insightful book!
Easy read! Good info! I enjoyed it thoroughly!

New book releases are free the first 24 hours. To know of new releases and dates for free downloads, please subscribe at www.TessaCason.com

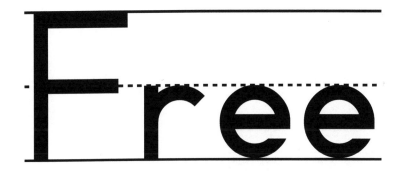

Muscle Testing
Obstacles and Helpful Hints

Tessa Cason, MA

Tessa Cason
5694 Mission Ctr. Rd. #602-213
San Diego, CA. 92108
www.TessaCason.com
Tessa@TessaCason.com

© Tessa Cason, 2023.

Table of Contents

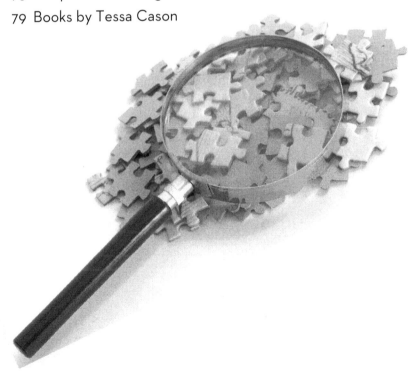

My Self-Discovery Journey

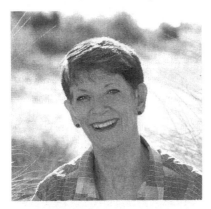

I was one of those baby boomer (born between 1946–1964, after the Second World War) in the 1970s that was searching for answers. We didn't have the internet, blogs, websites, YouTube videos to find answers. We had books, audiobooks on cassette tape, and sometimes, a live-in person seminar.

Cindy, another seeker, and I investigated anything that could increase our awareness of the new age dawning.

"Tessa, Donna Eden just returned from a workshop learning about energy. For $5, she will teach us what she learned. Let's go," said Cindy. And we did. One afternoon, a small group of us sat on her living room floor as Donna conducted her own mini workshop for us. I learned how to muscle test sitting on Donna Eden's living room floor more than forty years ago.

One day when Cindy and I were on a walk, I asked if she had heard of Louise Hay. She had not. "She is leading a class in La Jolla next week. No one wants to help gay people dying from AIDS. She does. Want to go?" And we went. It was eye-opening to learn that our thoughts could create dis-ease. In the 1970s, people didn't believe the food they ate impacted their health. The concept that our thoughts could impact our well-being was revolutionary for the time!

In 1980, I completed a thirteen week process called "Fischer-Hoffman: Getting a Loving Divorce from Mom and Dad." It was an intense thirteen weeks. Every week-end was spent journaling, reflecting, and processing my dysfunctional childhood. The facilitators for the process hosted weekly gatherings in their home for Siddha Yoga and Swami Muktananda. Halfway through the process, I started attending the weekly gatherings. Once I completed the program, I decided to visit the Siddha Yoga Center in upstate New York.

It was the summer of 1980, and the Catskills were beautiful, very peaceful, and the perfect place to find serenity. The purpose of the center was to provide a location where students could study the philosophy of Siddha Yoga. I lived in the ashram for two months taking classes, learning about Siddha Yoga, the self, and self-realization. Muktananda was in residence for a month while I was in the Catskills. I attended his nightly meetings.

My journey for personal growth led to Murrieta Hot Springs in Southern California. A group called Alive Polarity offered workshops to transform the self. Students lived at the retreat while attending their workshops. I completed two workshops, living at the retreat for fourteen weeks. We met six days a week, six to seven hours each day. It was as intense as going through boot camp.

In 1985, a new breakfast group was formed called The Inside Edge. We met once a week at 6 AM for breakfast and a speaker. I heard new authors, such as Brian Tracy, Mark Victor Hansen, Jack Canfield, Susan Jeffers, and many others after they had written their first book.

At this time, I was employed at The Learning Annex, assisting with hosting events. The Learning Annex was an education company that offered a wide range of classes with diverse topics. This is a short list of speakers I heard speak:

* Wayne Dyer
* James Redfield
* Dan Millman
* David Hawkins
* Deepak Chopra
* Marianne Williamson
* Melody Beattie
* Barbara Marx Hubbard
* Neale Donald Walsch
* Byron Katie
* Don Miguel Ruiz
* Richard Bach

In 1988, I attended a promo event for a new speaker on the lecture circuit, Tony Robbins. I returned for the weekend event, which included a firewalk. Without the internet in 1988, there were no YouTube videos or internet searches to pre-pare oneself for Tony or for walking on fire. Saying that *UPW, Unleash the Power Within*, was the most transformational event I have ever completed falls short of how spectacular and life changing UPW was.

The three-day event began on Friday. Throughout the first day, Tony had us do various exercises to prepare us for the firewalk. Around midnight, he marched the entire room of people to the parking lot.

As we approached the asphalt, we heard tribal drums beating, the crackling of logs burning and smelled the fiery embers. When the huge pile of wood came into view, we felt the blast of heat coming off the fire. Flames and sparks were shooting high into the air. The immediate thought one has is, *Really? I am going to walk across that? That's fire. It's hot, and it burns!*

Around 3 AM, everyone in the ballroom once again marched to the parking lot. We found rows of embers, ten feet long, with staff at each line. With the drums beating, excitement in the air, and everyone chanting, we lined up behind a row of coals.

When we reached the front of the line, a staff member determined if we were truly ready. They looked us in the eye, assessed our psychological readiness, looked at our body language, and told us to either go or get back in line because we were not ready.

At the end of the bed of coals, we were jumping for joy, excited, and a little in disbelief about what we just accomplished. It was an amazing experience, something you never forget. Thirty-five years later, I can still remember walking across red-hot coals and feeling triumphant as I celebrated the achievement.

After UPW, I completed every program and event Tony had, which included Date with Destiny and Mastery University. At

Mastery Universe, Tony had a thirty-five-foot firewalk along with the ten-foot bed of coals. After confidently walking the ten-foot bed of coals, I walked the thirty-five-foot, and then went back and did the ten-foot bed of coals again. It was fun!

After attending all of Tony's programs, earning several certifications, I volunteered to staff his events and helped with a dozen fire walks.

Another influential mentor was Caroline Myss. In the 1990s, I read and listened to all her books and lectures. I particularly like her work on Archetypes and have incorporated her work into my life coaching practice.

The journey of self-discovery is perpetual and ongoing. We are complex, exciting people who are constantly learning, evolving, and transforming. Having knowledge of who we are and where we want to go is key to our transformations. Staying the same, staying safe, staying inside our comfort zones and rut is boring.

Knowledge is the accumulation of information. Wisdom is the application of the knowledge. Once we have the knowledge of ourselves, we can apply that knowledge to become the best version of ourselves.

Starting a self-discovery journey in the late 1960s, I have gone through a number of different programs and acquired several certifications and degrees. In 1996, when life coaching was in its infancy, I established a life coaching practice. I utilize muscle-testing with each client and every session.

> Muscle-testing is a great tool for self-improvement and healing.

Chapter 1
Muscle Testing Technique
aka Kinesiology or Energy Testing

Muscle testing is a method in which we can converse with the subconscious mind as well as the body's nervous system and energy field.

TECHNIQUE

Any large muscle in the body can be utilized for testing. The arm may be one of the easiest to test. The following description is for the arm.

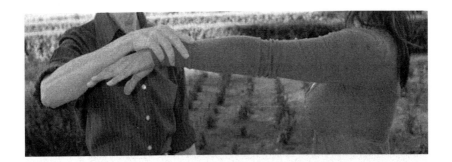

1. The testee (woman on right) lifts her arm directly in front of her shoulder, parallel with the ground, elbow straight, hand open, facing down.

2. The tester (woman on left) places her hand on or just above the wrist (towards the elbow) on the extended arm of the testee.

3. The tester tells the testee, "Resist," **then** applies downward pressure on the arm of the testee. The objective is not to overpower the arm with force. Applying a minimal amount of pressure will accomplish a more accurate answer than a forceful press.

4. The testee, when asked to "Resist," is to maintain the current arm position as pressure is exerted on their arm. The temptation of the testee is to lift the arm upward to counteract the downward pressure. Not good.

5. With a positive, **"yes,"** or **true statement**, the arm will **remain strong** as if locked in place.

6. With a negative, **"no,"** or **false statement**, the arm will be **weak and drop**.

ADDITIONAL COMMENTS

ALTERNATIVE ARM POSITIONING

Some testers like the arm at a 45 degree angle to the side, while others like it straight out to the side from the shoulder. If I am going to use the arm to ask a number of questions, the arm seems to tire more quickly when out to the side of the body.

TESTEE'S HAND

Testee's hand should be open, with fingers extending out. Some testees have a tendency to make a fist with their hand. This blocks energy from flowing freely. If the testee's hand is in a fist, ask them to open their hand and point their finger straight.

RESIST OR HOLD

Some testers prefer to ask the testee to "hold" instead of "resist." Either works. It is a matter of preference. The key is more about the timing of when to apply the pressure. The pressure is applied AFTER the testee is asked to hold or resist.

Chapter 2
The Physiology of Muscle Testing

With a positive or yes response, the arm remains strong. With a negative or no response, the arm is weakened. Okay...how does the muscle know?

The skeletal muscles are controlled by the nervous system. Electrical energy travels through the nervous system. When pressure is applied to the muscle in muscle testing, the muscle will either test strong or weak, depending on whether the energy is able to flow unobstructed through the nervous system.

Electrical energy that is not able to flow freely, blocked energy, is experienced as weakness by the nervous system, thus weakening the muscle. If the "answer" to the question is "no" or a substance that is being tested is detrimental, it will block the electrical energy in the body. As a result, the muscle will test weak. If the answer is "yes" or a substance is beneficial, the muscle will test strong.

Our body's electrical activity reveals a great deal about our health and well-being. An EKG measures the electrical activity of the heart which tells us about the health of the heart. An EEG measures the electrical activity of the brain. Brain death is when there is no activity on the EEG.

Different Systems in the Body

The circulatory system moves blood throughout the body. The nervous system is a vast network of nerves that sends electrical signals throughout the body. And the respiratory system brings air into and out of the lungs. But what about energy? What system is responsible for generating and moving energy in the body? The circulatory system has arteries and veins, the nervous system has nerves, and the respiratory system uses blood to supply air to the cells of the body. But, what about energy?

In Chinese philosophy, energy is called "chi," (also known as qi, prana, and life force in other cultures). Chi flows through our bodies and is impacted by every thought we think, every word we speak, every action we take, and every belief we hold.

Traditional Chinese Medicine, thousands of years ago, mapped out the energy pathways in the physical body. These pathways are called meridians and are paths in which energy travels throughout the body. Think super highway, rivers, and streams.

When blood and oxygen are able to flow unobstructed, the body is healthy. If there are any restrictions to blood or oxygen flow, illness will result. When an accident happens on a super highway, the flow of traffic is impacted. When rivers and streams become polluted with debris, water stops flowing.

When energy is able to flow freely, unobstructed, the body is healthy. Dis-ease happens when the energy is blocked. Every breath, emotion, and thought reflects the state and quality of our chi. Energy can become blocked by our thoughts, speech, actions, and beliefs as well as stress, injury, and trauma.

When we muscle test, we are testing the energy that flows along the meridians in the physical body.

Chinese Meridians

Yang (front edge)

inner surface = yin

lungs
pericardium
heart

(palm)

Yin (back edge)

outer surface = yang

small intestine
lymphatic system
large intestine

(knuckles)

Yang (front edge)

Chapter 3
Ten Obstacles to Successful Muscle Testing

Even though muscle testing is an easy technique to learn, it is a complicated skill to master. It requires a lot of practice on a diverse number of people asking a variety of questions. If the technique is not perfected, the answers are questionable.

One client I had, Mia, when pressure was applied, and the answer was a "no," the arm dropped to her side. The first time it happened, I asked if she dropped her arm on purpose. She said she hadn't. She was the easiest to test. Another client, Jim, was my most difficult client to muscle test. We both had to be very perceptive of the smallest of movement in his arm. One of my favorite clients was Barbara. As soon as a question was asked, before I applied pressure, she verbalized the answer. The first time she did, a surprised me asked how she knew. "I can feel my arm immediately become very heavy and it's difficult to hold up or it becomes strong as a steel rod," she replied.

A women's group asked if I would give a demonstration at one of their monthly meetings. I accepted the invitation. As I was describing the technique, Jill jumped up to be my volunteer. Before I could begin she said, "I don't believe in muscle testing nor do I think I can be muscle tested." A stunning way to begin a demonstration. I responded, "There will always be a first person I am not able to muscle test."

Jill's arm provided clear responses to pressure applied to her arm. "You are using thirty-three and one-third more pressure on the yes than you are on the no," she said with some fluster. Apparently, this was normal behave from Jill. Another woman in the group responded, "Jill, we all saw her apply less pressure for the no response. She did not use more muscle on the no response. She actually used less."

My response to the doubting Jill was the "zipper." Knowing this would intrigue her, hesitantly I said, "Jill, there is one way to know whether you can be muscle tested. It's called the zipper. Would you like to see whether you can be unzipped?" She was hooked! I explained the "zipper," (see #6 of helpful hints). I waved my hand downward 2" in front of her body. Before muscle testing her, I asked her to watch my bicep to determine how much energy I was exerting. When I know an answer will be no, I will use one finger to apply the pressure.

The look on Jill's face was priceless when one finger was able to drop her arm down to her side. Without a respond, Jill returned to her seat. I asked if she wanted to be zipped back up. Still, without saying anything, she stood back in front of me. I followed suit, did not say a word, but zipped her back up, muscle tested she was strong again. She, then, returned to her seat, all without uttering a word.

Jill was not my first person I could not muscle test. Actually, I still have not had someone I could not muscle test. Knowing how to muscle test correctly and how to overcome difficulties in muscle testing, I have been able to muscle test everyone I have worked with.

DEHYDRATION

Before I begin this section on the obstacles to muscle testing successfully, I would like to mention dehydration. In some of the literature you will read and some of the teacher that teach muscle testing, they might mention the reason the tester cannot muscle test correctly is because the tester is dehydrated. If one is dehydrated, drinking a glass or two of water will not hydrate a person and then they are able to accurately muscle test someone.

Dehydration affects millions of people in the United States. 75% of Americans are chronically dehydrated. A survey of 3,003 Americans found that 75% likely had a net fluid loss, resulting in chronic dehydration. Does that mean 75% of Americans will have difficulty muscle testing? No. I have not found dehydration to be a factor in muscle testing.

I am one of those 75% than is chronically dehydrated. Here is a way in which to know if you are dehydrated. Place your hand on a flat surface. Pinch the back of your hand and release the flesh. If the skin snap backs to your hand, you are hydrated. If it slowly eases back to the hand, you are dehydrated.

TEN OBSTACLES

1. Muscle testing is not a competition. It is not a test of strength of the muscle, but rather the flow of energy.

2. It is a necessity that the tester be someone that (1) calibrates the same as, or above, that of the testee, on David Hawkins' Map of Consciousness (*Power vs. Force: The Hidden Determinants of Human Behavior*) or (2) is in the higher altitudes,

250 or higher, on the Map. (See page 65, Chapter 9 – Map of Consciousness for more information.)

DAVID HAWKINS' MAP OF CONSCIOUSNESS

Levels of Conscious

Level	Log
[Higher Altitudes]	
Enlightenment	700-1000
Peace	600
Joy	540
Love	500
Reason	400
Acceptance	350
Willingness	310
Neutrality	250
[Lower Altitudes]	
Courage	200
Pride	175
Anger	150
Desire	125
Fear	100
Grief	75
Apathy	50
Guilt	30
Shame	20

© David R. Hawkins, *Power vs. Force: The Hidden Determinant of Human Behavior*

3. Wording of the question or statement is <u>critical</u>. Be as **specific as possible**. Ask one thing at a time. (See page 47, Chapter 7 - Asking Questions.)

4. Always begin testing with asking the testee to "Resist." If the arm is strong, proceed to asking the body for a "yes" and a "no" response. (If the arm is weak, see #5.)

* Have the testee says, "Yes," then test the arm. The arm should remain strong.

* Have the testee says "No," then test the arm. The arm should drop and/or dip.

* Have the testee say, "My name is <u>(fill in their own name)</u>," then test. The arm should stay strong.

* Have the testee say, "My name is <u>(a name not their own)</u>," then test. The arm should drop.

If, on any of the above, the arm does the opposite, some of the other Obstacles and/or Helpful Hints might provide reasons and possible solutions.

5. When the muscle is not giving a clear, strong yes, thump the thymus. The thymus is beneath the breastbone, about a hand's width below the throat. Thump about 25 times.

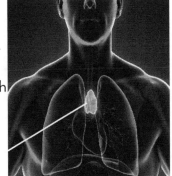

Thymus Gland

6. Tester and testee should not make eye contact with each other. With eye contact, the answer would be "our" energy instead of the "testee's" energy.

7. Our intuition is accurate when we are in present time. When in present time, it is possible that the tester will know the answer before applying pressure on the muscle. Don't make assumptions or guess. Test for the answer.

8. The tester must be in present time. When we are not in present time, we are either in the past or the future, our regrets or our worries, or our anger or our fear. If the tester is not in present time, the testing response will be filtered through the tester's "dirty lenses."

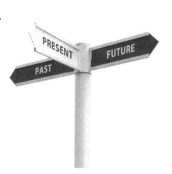

9. It is possible when muscle testing the muscle/arm will stay strong for a "no" and weak for a "yes." This is called "reversed" or "reversal." The energy is actually flowing in the opposite direction. There are a number of reasons this can happen. One of the main reasons I have discovered is fear. In Chinese medicine, the kidney meridian is associated with fear. When someone is reversed, I have found that the kidney meridian is flowing in the wrong direction.

There are several exercises one can do to reverse the reversal, but as soon as the fear resurfaces, the individual goes back into reversal.

Fear has an electrical current to it. Two stones, **Rutilated Quartz** and **Hematite** have electrical currents to them and can switch someone in reversal. These two gemstones, along with **Garnet** and **Chrysocolla**, greatly enhance an individual who has a tendency to go into reversal and/or is dealing with fear. Putting these four gemstones in a pouch and having a client put them in a pocket during a session is useful for those that have a tendency to go into reversal.

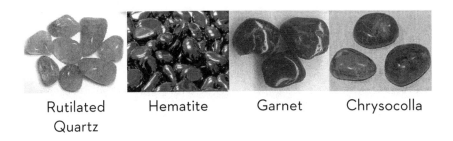

Rutilated   Hematite   Garnet   Chrysocolla
Quartz

I worked with several children that were diagnosed with Attention-deficit/hyperactivity disorder (ADHD). All the ADHD children I worked with were reversed. Once they had a pouch of stones in their pockets, they tested correctly. Each child asked for a pouch of the stones. Parents reported back that they (the parents) and the child noticed the difference in the child when they had the pouch of stones with them. They were not hyper, but acted normally.

Some parents found jewelry with one or more of the stones that the children would wear. One ten-year old little girl loved her Hermatite necklace. Rachael was so excited to receive her necklace at her next appointment, she ran into my office, gave me a hug, and told me how wonderful her life had been since wearing the necklace and how normal she felt. "I feel just like the other kids. Since I act like them, they don't make fun of me anymore." She was beaming as were her parents.

The children became mindful of their behavior with and without the pouch of stones. One little boy, Jeffrey, when he noticed a basket full of pouches I had in my office, he asked, "Since you have so many, can I have another pouch?" He did not want to be without. He selected a blue pouch since blue was his favorite color.

10. The tester must be an "open vessel."

* Without passing judgment of any answer the testee's body provides. The tester needs to remain objective and nonjudgemental.

* Without an expectation of failure on the part of the tester. A tester thinking "I can't do this" will have less chance of being successful.

 * Without any expectation or desired outcome of a specific answer. The objective is to determine the testee's truth rather than the tester being "right."

I had a client/student, Jay, that after muscle testing himself would then ask me to muscle test him with the same question. Many times, the answers differed. For Jay, he had to add a second step to his muscle testing himself. After the initial request, he had to follow up with a second question, "Am I influencing the answer?"

I was super surprised that his body told him he was! Jay had to ask this second question after multiple questions for many years until he was able to detach from the answer.

Chapter 4
Ten Helpful Hints

Muscle testing was one of my favorite classes to teach. Of all the classes I taught, this class had the most variety of people with diversity ages, backgrounds, belief systems, and education levels. Sixty-year old grandmothers, businessmen, young adults, and everything in between populated the classes.

Having such an assortment of participants provided a great opportunity for the students to practice muscle testing on someone outside their normal sphere of friends and acquaintances. We have a tendency to surround ourselves with others that are much like ourselves. Every student, all beginners and strangers to each other, were able to practice muscle testing with someone very different from themselves as well as unknown to them.

Sometimes it is easier to begin learning the skill with someone you do not know. This reduces your expectations of what the answer should be or what you want it to be. But, if you have the belief you could fail and look stupid in front of someone you don't know, this could make it more difficult.

Joy was an interesting student. She arrived early, listened closely to the instruction, and failed miserably. "I just can't do it. I am a failure. I will never learn how to muscle test correctly. I really wanted to master this skill," she mumbled through her tears at the break.

Ah, I thought. *Perfect student to teach about expectations and beliefs that interfere with being successful learning this skill.*

After the break, I asked how many people felt as Joy did that they would never be able to master the skill of muscle testing. In every class, at least half of the participants responded they felt very much like Joy did. As a class, we explored the beliefs that complicated their learning the new skill. Following the discussion, we eliminated the unhelpful beliefs using EFT Tapping, Emotional Freedom Technique. EFT is a method that easily eliminated dysfunctional beliefs on a subconscious level.

It would be helpful for you to contempt the beliefs you have about learning and mastering a new skill. On my website: www. TessaCason.com, I have instructions on how to tap.

Ten Helpful Hints

1. Always ask the body for permission to muscle test. "Do I have permission to muscle test _____?" then apply pressure to the arm. If the answer is "no," stop. Even if the person gives you verbal permission, stop. This is an invasion of privacy and the results may be compromised and thus, not valid.

2. Right side of the body represents male energy, whereas the left side represents female energy. Male energy is dominant... i.e. likes to be right, whereas the female energy is receptive. Thus, the tester might want to consider using the left side to begin. If the left side fatigues, switch to the right side.

3. Can a tester determine and/or influence the answer for a testee? If the tester:

1) is consistent with the amount of pressure they apply,

2) does not make eye contact,

3) is in present time,

4) asks the body for permission, and

5) calibrates higher than the testee on the Map of Consciousness or calibrates in the higher altitudes on the Map,

then the response will solely be that of the testee. If any of the above are not adhered to, if the testee or tester are reversed, then the answers will lack validity.

4. Do not ask the question: "Is this for my highest and best good." We learn from pain and struggle, thus pain and struggle could be for our highest and best good.

> # Is this for my highest and best good?
>
> # Can you learn without pain and struggle?

5. Muscle testing is **not** "predictive." Only the "present," the "now" exists, only "now" can be muscle tested.

6. The immediate response of someone experiencing muscle testing for the first time usually is the following: "This is a trick!" or "You are using more energy on the 'no' than you are on the 'yes'." This is when I like to introduce the zipper.

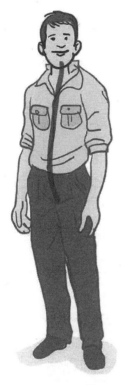

* The central meridian, in Chinese medicine, runs straight up the front of the body, from the pubic bone to the bottom lip. If this meridian is not flowing up, it weakens the muscle being tested.

HOW TO UNZIP

* Muscle test the testee. Response should be strong.

* Then, run your hand down the front of their body, about 2 - 3" in front of the body (and **not touching the body**), starting at the lip down to the pubic bone.

* Retest the muscle. It will now be weak.

* Remember to zip back up! Starting at the pubic bone, about 2 - 3" in front of the body (and **not touching the body**), run your hand up to the lips.

7. It is possible to surrogate test for another person or an animal that may not be present or able to be tested. It is not necessary to actually be in physical touch or proximity to the one being surrogate tested.

* Very important: Muscle-testing, first ask for permission. "Do we have permission to ask questions for/about (name of person or animal)?"

* If the answer is "no," stop. If you continued, it would be a violation of privacy and the accuracy of the questions could be compromised. Even if the person gives a verbal "yes," still stop.

* If the answer is "yes," the testee "assumes" that person's or animal's identity. Have the testee say, "My name is (name of the person or animal)." The response should be a "yes."

* Have the testee say, "My name is (have them say their real name)." The response should be "no." Proceed with the questioning.

Note from Tessa: One of my cats was anemic. He had an allergic reaction to Advantage, a topical medication to rid an animal of fleas. Fleas were sucking all his blood. With every treatment the vet suggested for his anemia, I muscle-tested to determine if it would be safe as well as effective for him. The vet allowed me to use her as the surrogate for my cat.

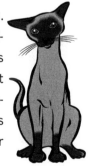

8. Using David Hawkins' Map of Consciousness, it is beneficial to calibrate those things in our life that we are involved with and/or want to know how it could possibly impact our life. This includes such things as bodyworkers, teachers, chiropractors, seminars, companies, websites, programs, books, information, and/or our "truths."

Example: I had a client that calibrated around 100 – 125 when she began working with me. As she continued to process her unhealthy, dysfunctional beliefs, she was able to maintain the higher altitudes of 250+. She enjoyed her massages. One day she commented that she wasn't enjoying her massages as much as she once did. 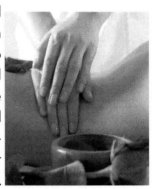 She wanted to calibrate the masseuse when she was working on her and where she (my client) calibrated as a result of using this masseuse. The masseuse calibrated lower than where my client calibrated. My client's calibration dropped as a result of getting a massage from this masseuse.

9. When testing, it is possible to know from the softness of a "yes," when the muscle would test "no." Example: "Day in and day out, this individual is in present time at least 65% of the time" and the muscle tests strong. "70%" and the response is a little soft. "71%" and the muscle is weak.

10. As with any new skill, practice, practice, practice. The more people you can practice with, the better able you are to "detect" a "no." With some people, the "no" is not easily discernible.

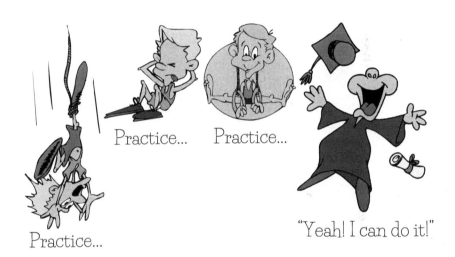

Practice...

Practice...

Practice...

"Yeah! I can do it!"

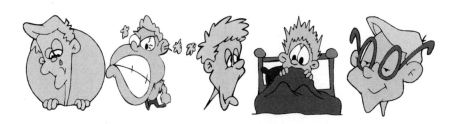

Which one of these guys would
you want testing you?

Which one are you
when you are testing?

Chapter 5
Value of Mastering Self-Muscle Testing

The first advantage of learning self-muscle testing is that you are the only one needed to participant in this activity. Not partner required!

The primary reason is to be able to access our own body's infinite wisdom. It is a way in which we can discover dysfunctional beliefs in the subconscious, determine food allergies, or improve our decisions.

A few days ago, I became very ill, nauseous, and had a headache. I thought back to what transpired throughout the day and started muscle testing to determine the cause of feeling ill. When I asked about a new frying pan, the answer tested positive. The coating on the frying pan was toxic for my body.

I particularly appreciate the ability to muscle test when I am trying to discern if what I am feeling is me or someone else. I am not a donut lover, but I have a client that is. I went through several "donut cravings" until I realized I could ask if the cravings were my cravings or my clients. Great tool to find the truth.

Most useful, though, I think is being able to find a bottom line to dysfunctional beliefs. Before sliding into frustration or depression, I use muscle testing to determine the beliefs that cause me to be out of synch with myself and/or the world around me.

The list is long of the values to mastering how to muscle test ourselves.

Chapter 6
Seven Self-Muscle Testing Techniques

Muscle testing yourself could be one of the most significant tools and skills you can learn for yourself. There are a number of different ways you can muscle test yourself. One of these may work for you:

BENT ELBOW

I broke my elbow and needed to be able to muscle test myself. My go-to technique was the extended arm. With a broken elbow, I was not able to extend my arm. I came up with this technique and now this is my favorite go-to technique for muscle testing myself!

* Bend your left arm. Bring the hand up toward the shoulder.

* Place your right hand or fist on your left wrist.

* Ask: "Show me a yes." The arm should remain strong and closed.

* Ask: "Show me a no." The arm should do the **opposite of the yes,** open.

This is my "yes" and "no" responses. For one of my clients, it is the opposite. For her "yes," the arm opens and for her "no," the arm remains closed.

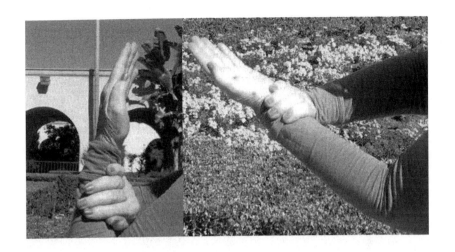

Leaning Forward and Backwards/Sway

* Standing upright, feet shoulder width apart or whatever is comfortable, arms hanging at your side or crossed in front of your chest.

* Ask: "Show me a yes." More likely, your body will lean forward.

* Ask: "Show me a no." More likely, your body will lean backwards.

I have a friend that uses his chair. It's a little wobbly. His body would tilt, lean, or fall to the right for a "yes" and to the left for a "no."

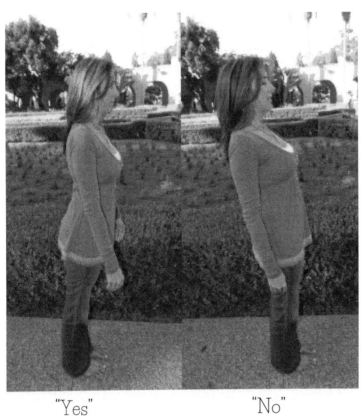

"Yes"   "No"

SMOOTH AND STICKY

* Rub the pad of your index finger on the left hand over the top of the left hand's thumbnail.

* Ask: "Show me a yes response." Usually this is a smooth response and the finger glides easily across the thumbnail.

* Ask: "Show me a no response." Usually the finger will get stuck, making it very difficult to rub the finger across the thumbnail.

* Sometimes, the answers are reversed. The "yes" response is sticky and the "no" response is smooth.

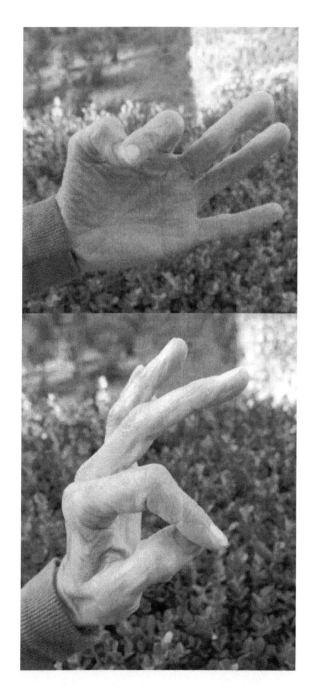

Thumb/Little Finger Loop

* Bring the thumb and little finger together on your left hand.

* Place the thumb and index finger on the right hand inside the left hand's thumb and ring/little finger loop.

* Holding the left fingers closed, ask: "Show me a yes." With the thumb and index fingers on your right hand *apply pressure against* the left finger's thumb and little finger by opening the fingers like scissors. The left fingers should remain closed or separate a tad bit.

* Ask: "Show me a no." With the right hand's thumb and index finger, apply pressure against the left hand's thumb and little finger. This time the fingers on the left hand should separate.

* It is necessary to apply the same amount of pressure when asking all your questions.

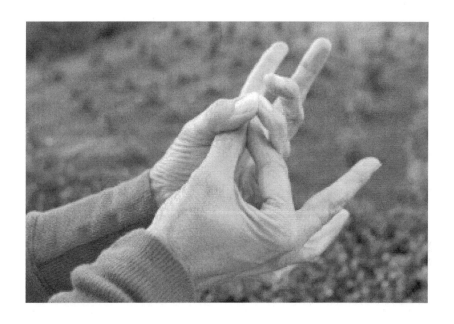

Double Loops

* Bring the thumb and the middle fingers together on the left hand to form a loop.

* With the right hand, bring the thumb and the middle fingers together so that they interlock between the left hand's finger loop.

* Ask: "Show me a yes response," and pull the fingers on the right hand against the point at which the two fingers on the left hand meet. Both sets of rings should stay together.

* Ask: "Show me a no response." Apply pressure against the fingers on the left hand with the right hand's fingers. With a no response, the right hand fingers should slip through the left hand finger's loop.

* It is necessary to apply the same amount of pressure when asking all your questions.

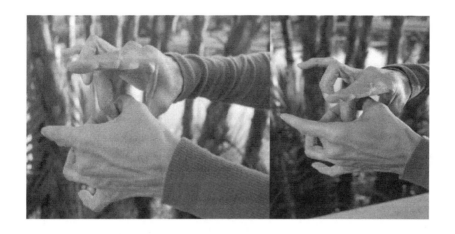

Two Finger Loop with One Finger Tester

* Bring the thumb together with either the index or middle finger on the left hand.

* Put the index finger on the right hand inside the loop.

* Ask: "Show me a yes response" and with the index finger on the right side, apply pressure against the junction where the thumb and index/middle finger on the left hand come together. The loop should stay together.

* Ask: "Show me a no response." Apply pressure against the junction where the thumb and index/middle finger on the left hand come together. The index finger on the right hand should slip through the left hand's fingers loop.

* It is necessary to apply the same amount of pressure when asking all your questions.

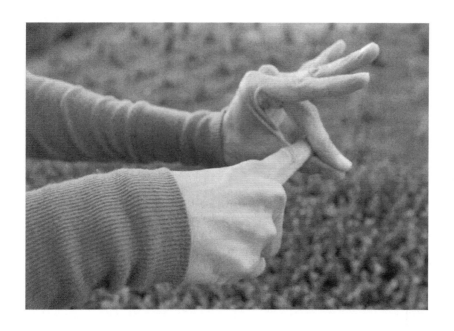

FULL ARM PRESS

* Same as the two person muscle-testing. Put your left arm straight out in front of you, parallel to the ground.

* Place your right hand on your left arm, somewhere between the elbow and the wrist.

* Ask: "Show me a yes response" and apply pressure to your left arm. The arm should stay strong, feeling no stress in the shoulder joint.

* Ask: "Show me a no response." Apply the same amount of pressure at the same location to the left arm. The arm will be weak. You will feel stress in the shoulder joint if you try to resist.

* It is important that you apply the same amount of pressure each time you ask a question.

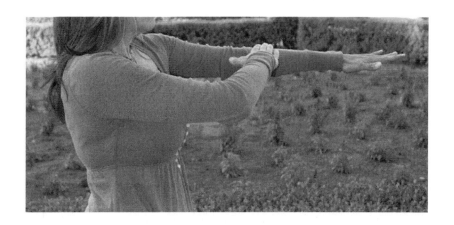

Chapter 7
Eight Rules When Asking Questions

Learning and mastering how to ask questions is the most difficult aspect of muscle testing. In comparison, perfecting the technique is a hundred times easier than becoming skillful at wording questions.

There are two different thoughts of "asking question." I had one mentor that preferred to make a statement versus a question. The difference between a statement and question are the arrangement of the first several words.

This job opportunity is the right decision for me at this time.

Is this job opportunity the right decision for me at this time?

It is a matter of prefers. Both are correct. Whether you prefer a statement or question, there are eight "rules" to keep in mind when practicing and refining the skill of asking questions.

1. BE AS SPECIFIC AND CLEAR AS POSSIBLE.

An ambiguous question could result in a vague, puzzling answer or a response that does not make sense. For example: "Did you see the film last weekend?" Other than the weekend, the question is fuzzy. What film? A movie on tv or at a cinema? A more specific question would be: "Did you see the latest superhero movie at the cinema last week-end?"

"Why am I unhappy and sad?" This inquiry is undefined, hazy, and clouded in confusion.

A more specific and clear question would be: "Is part or all of the reason I am unhappy have to do with my health?" If the answer is no, move on to another aspect of possibly being unhappy.

"If part or all of the reason I am unhappy and sad at this time have to do with my personal relationships?" If the answer is yes, then the questions can be more specific, asking one relationship at a time.
* "Friends?"
* "Family?"
* "Spouse?"
* "Coworkers?"

Murky, weird, and confounding questions result in cloaked, shaded, and baffling answers.

2. ASKING QUESTIONS IS LIKE MOVING DOWN A FUNNEL WITH EACH LEVEL BECOMING MORE SPECIFIC.

Continuing to use the example from rule #1:

The broad question is: "Is part or all of the reason I am unhappy have to do with my health?"

Narrowing down the areas of our lives would be the next step down in the funnel. Those areas could be:

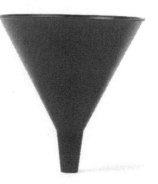

* Relationships
* Employment
* Career
* Finances
* Self-care
* Home environment
* Personal development
* Spiritually

Narrowing the specific area of our unhappiness, takes us further down the funnel.

After determining that "relationships" contributed to some or all of your unhappiness, the next step would be which sort of relationship:

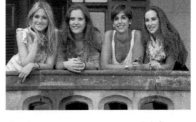

* Spouse
* Parents
* Children
* Friendships
* Coworkers

Still moving down the funnel, the next step could be more details about the different aspect of the relationship. Maybe you determined which friendship was impacting your happiness. Concerns on your part could be:

* They don't create any time to get together.
* They aren't supporting my efforts to improve my life.
* They don't offer the support I need while going through a difficult patch in my life.

Asking questions is like moving down a funnel from broad brush strokes to finite lines.

3. ONLY ASK ONE ASPECT OF A QUESTION AT A TIME.

Question: Is my issue with George about disliking him personally or professionally?

When the word "or" is included in the question, it implies one or the other. If you *know* you dislike George personally, you might be confused when the answer to your inquiry is "no," the issue with George is not about disliking him personally or professionally. But you so dislike him personally!

The way in which we can determine if both are true is to include the word "and." The question then becomes, "Is my issue with George about disliking him personally and/or professionally?" After discerning a "yes" response, then if more clarity is needed, you ask: "Both personally and professionally?"

4. BE NEUTRAL.

Really wanting an answer to be "Yes" or "No" can influence the answer.

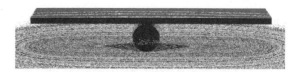

During one of my muscle testing classes, one of the students decided that he would test himself to determine where he calibrated on the Map of Consciousness. When he calibrated himself at "Enlightenment," the highest calibration on the map, I started laughing.

He turned toward me, smiled, and said, "Maybe I wasn't being neutral."

5. Use "Should" Questions Sparingly.

In class, a student asked herself a question: *Should I break up with my boyfriend?* When the arm stayed strong, which indicated a "Yes" response, she looked at me with dismay. "But, I don't want to break up with my boyfriend," she said. "Why did it tell me to break up with him?"

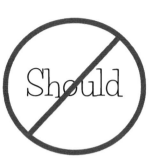

This was a great teaching example for the whole class on using "should" in the question.

I asked the student, "What do you really want to know?"

She pondered the question for a few minutes then responded, "I guess I'm wanting to know if I am going to get my heart broken. If I break up with him before that happens, my heart won't get broken."

"Do you like this guy?"

"I do. Probably more than any other guy I have dated. That's why I think I should break up with him before he ends the relationship."

I was left confused by her logic. It certainly wasn't sound and seemed as if she was making lots of assumptions.

I asked, "If you like the guy and you broke up with him, wouldn't that break your heart?"

"I guess it would. I don't want to get hurt."

Maybe the question isn't about breaking up. You might want to explore the reasons why you think he might end the relationship or the reasons why you want to give up a relationship that is fulfilling or maybe what your fears are in a relationship that you enjoy."

Another student asked, "How could she have worded the question?"

A discussion followed with the students, each offering how she could ask what she really wanted to know.

6. CONSIDER USING A RATING SCALE OF 1–10.

Example:

You: I'm considering changing companies. I've been offered a position with another company. I would be doing the same job that I am currently doing in HR. The industry is different, more or less, but the responsibilities are the same.

Tessa: Would this be a lateral move?

You: Yes.

Tessa: What is your question?

You: Well, would it be beneficial to change jobs?

Tessa: Beneficial financially, work conditions, work environment, or emotionally?

You: All of the above.

Tessa: Rank each job, current and potential, on a scale of 1–10, based on each of the benefits. On a scale of 1–10, with 1 being the lowest, how fulfilling would this new job be?

Example:

You: I want to know if my health will improve by pursuing this treatment.

Tessa: What about asking on a scale of 1–10: If I pursue this treatment, how beneficial would the treatment be for my physical health?

Example:

You: I want to know if this supplement is beneficial for my health.

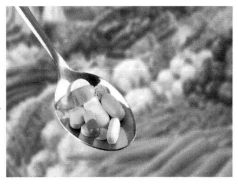

Tessa: You can ask on a scale of 1–10: How beneficial would a supplement be for the improvement of my health?

Besides supplements, we can rate different therapists, programs, and/or books, in regard to how beneficial they might be for our health, personal growth, or whatever the objective might be.

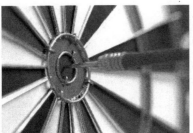

7. WORDING OF A QUESTION COULD DETERMINE THE VALIDITY AND ACCURACY OF AN ANSWER.

Let's look more in-depth at an inquiry that you might have. Remember:

1) Wording is critical
2) Be as specific as possible
3) Singularly focused

Example:

Let's say you ask the question: Should I move cross country to live with my boyfriend?

The answer that you received was a "Yes." You moved cross country. Spent all your savings moving and now have a zero balance in your bank accounts. After a month of looking for a job, you are still unemployed, and your boyfriend ends the relationship, asking you to move out.

You have no place to live, no income to afford another place to live, and no means of returning home. Yikes! "But...when I tested, the answer was a yes!"

1) "Should I," you asked. If you have a belief that the only way you can learn is through pain and struggle, you probably learned a lot from this experience!

2) This question has multiple parts to it.
    a) Move cross country
    b) Live with my boyfriend

When asking questions, it is best to be
as singularly focused as possible.

Let's re-examine this question: Should I move cross country to live with my boyfriend?

Tessa: What is the objective, goal, or intent of your question?

You: To know if I would be happy moving cross country to live with my boyfriend.

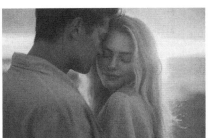

T: Are there other factors involved in this inquiry?

Y: Well, yes. It is a necessity for me to get a job as quickly as possible. My boyfriend doesn't want to support me. He wants me to share the expenses. It will take most, if not all, of the money that I have to move. I will need to get a job as soon as possible.

T: Have you looked into how easy this might be?

Y: Yes. I've looked in the paper and online.

T: Have you spent an extended period of time with your boy-friend, in his space?

Y: Yes. For our vacations, I usually fly cross country to spend time with him. The longest I have stayed was for two weeks. Everything worked out well.

T: Define "happy".

Y: Happy. Well, I do understand that no relationship is trouble-free. All relationships will have problems. When they happen, it is important to negotiate a solution.

T: Have the two of you had to negotiate anything in the past?

Y: Yes.

T: And how did that go?

Y: It was interesting. He wanted his way, typical man, you know. He pouted, got angry, and would not talk to me until I finally gave in.

T: Does that work for you?

Y: Well, sometimes. I realize that I need to compromise. I can't always have my way.

T: Is marriage important to you?

Y: Yes.

T: And for him?

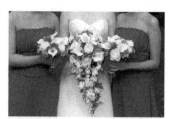

Y: It is not as important to him as it is to me. He's still thinking about whether he wants to be married.

T: This is okay with you that he doesn't know if he ever wants to marry?

Y: Yes. I think, well...I am hoping that once we live together for a while, he will not want to spend the rest of his life without me. Wishful thinking, I know. My eyes are wide open.

T: Define for me again the object of your inquiry?

Y: I can see that has changed. I would like to know if it is worth the gamble to move cross country and set up house with this man.

T: Everything is a risk and a gamble in life.

Y: Okay. Not definite enough.

T: Can you break your inquiry down into categories?

Y: Actually, I can. One has to do with finding a job and the monetary arena. The other is the relationship.

T: Which is the most important?

Y: That's a toughie. It is important to him that I pay half, pay my share. He doesn't want to support me. Moving cross country will drain all my funds. The relationship is equally as important.

T: Which is primary? Would you be looking for a job in that area if he were not living there?

Y: No. So, I need to determine if the relationship is good enough for me to leave behind everything I have here.

T: Good enough?

Y: Satisfying? Fulfilling? Worthwhile?

T: How about thinking more long-term, more workable, do-able, feasible, or viable?

Y: Okay. I get ya. I'm thinking more emotionally. You are thinking more practically. My head is up in the clouds. You have your feet on the ground.

T: Which is more important to you?

Y: Actually, more practical. Feet on the ground would be best. When my head is up in the clouds, it is difficult to see reality.

T: So, what is the real need? What is your objective now?

Y: I need to know if this relationship is strong enough to endure the everyday stresses of life.

T: The relationship? You or him?

Y: There is a difference, isn't there. Okay. Each of us in this relationship, with each other.

T: Anything else? Any other objectives? Any other needs?

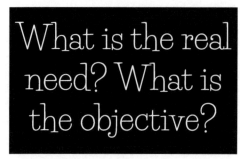
What is the real need? What is the objective?

Y: I guess, I would like to know if we do live together, will he get bored or will he want us to be together for a lifetime? Rather than assuming that he will feel as I hope he would feel, it might be better if I knew before I moved. I have been hesitant to ask him.

Now, I see it is better to deal with reality—what is real rather than make-believe or what I hope will be. It is my responsibility to take care of myself and not assume that everyone else will also have the same objective to take care of me.

T: Well stated. This can be your intent with this inquiry. The intent can be that you are responsible for yourself, your well-being, and your happiness.

You stated earlier your need. You stated that you needed to know if this relationship is strong enough to endure the everyday stresses of life. Your objective then is to make the wisest decision at this time with the information that you can gather.

Y: Sounds good to me.

T: Let's make a list of the questions now.

Y: Okay.

1. Living together under the same roof, this relationship can comfortably handle the stresses of everyday life. (You can add: "To a level of five or higher.")

2. Living together under the same roof, I can comfortably handle the stresses of everyday life, with this man to a level of five or higher."

3. We can successfully negotiate the stresses of everyday life and conflicts with each other.

4. Our styles of handling conflict are compatible with each other.

5. Currently, our styles of handling money are compatible with each other.

There are certainly many more questions that can be asked in regard to this question.

8. THERE IS A REASON THAT WE ASK THE QUESTIONS WE DO. THE REASONS ARE OUR OBJECTIVES.

It is important to know the objective when asking questions. Vague, unclear questions with inconclusive answers will have you thinking that you are unable to muscle test. The issue may not be your technique. The issue may be the wording of your inquiry!

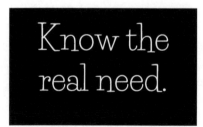

Know the
real need.

Conclusion:

It is an art and skill to learn how to word questions for muscle testing.

A friend in college was a mystery shopper for Jack in the Box drive-thru restaurants. He asked if I wanted to be a mystery shopper. (A mystery shopper is a consumer, just like everyone else. The store employees do not know that they are being evaluated. That's the mystery part.)

When I turned in my first shop, I said the hamburger was good. My friend called me into his office and said, "Good?"

"Yes," I answered.

"Wrong. Were the tomatoes fresh, was the lettuce crisp, was the bun warm, was there enough sauce on the bun?"

"Oh, more details."

> If our questions are vague, it will be difficult to know if the answers we receive are correct. The more details, the more specific and focused the question, the crisper the answers will be.

Chapter 8
Muscle Testing for Supplements

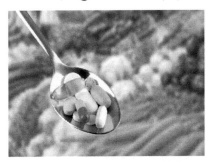

When I muscle test for supplements, I am very specific.

"Would this supplement be beneficial **at this time**, for the im-**provement of my health**, to a level of **8, 9, or 10?**"

"At this time." A supplement might have been beneficial last year or maybe in the future. I want to know if the supplement will be beneficial NOW.

"For the improvement of my health." If something is only going to maintain my health, I may not take the supplement. I had a gas leak in my home for 850 days, 2½ years. Part of getting well required ingesting 100+ supplements daily. Now I prefer liquid to pills and find it difficult to take lots of pills on a daily bases.

"To a level of 8, 9, or 10." If a supplement is only going to im-prove my health to a level of 1 - 5, I may not take the supple-ment. 6 or 7, I will strongly consider. To a level of 8, 9, or 10... my body is indicating this supplement will definitely improve my health. I will take the supplement.

Levels of Consciousness

[Higher Altitudes]

Enlighten-ment	700-1000
Peace	600
Joy	540
Love	500
Reason	400
Acceptance	350
Willingness	310
Neutrality	250

[Lower Altitudes]

Courage	200
Pride	175
Anger	150
Desire	125
Fear	100
Grief	75
Apathy	50
Guilt	30
Shame	20

© *David R. Hawkins, Power vs. Force, The Hidden Determinants of Human Behavior, 1995, 1998, 2004, 2012.*

Chapter 9
David Hawkins' Map of Consciousness

The Map of Consciousness (MOC) is a valuable tool. Our lives can be enhanced when we calibrate the people, teachers, books, learning institutions, health practice, etc on the Map of Consciousness.

The Map was developed by David Hawkins and introduced in his book *Power vs Force: The Hidden Determinant of Human Behavior*. It illustrates and outlines the levels of human consciousness. Twenty years of research involving millions of calibrations on thousands of test subjects of all ages, personality types, and all walks of life went into developing the Map of Consciousness.

With the Map, there is a lower altitude and a higher altitude. When we are in the lower altitudes, we are influenced by that level of consciousness whether that be fear, anger, or courage. Once we are able to maintain Neutrality, 250, we are in control of our lives. Anything less, 249 and lower, the emotion of that level is in charge.

At Neutrality (250), we learn not to take or make everything personal. When we are Willing (310) and Accepting (350), we open up new avenues of well-being.

"Love heals all." The Love at 500 on the Map is the love that heals even though some want to believe it is romantic love that heals (which it is not).

When we are in the higher altitudes, 250 or higher, we are able to objectively evaluate. The lenses through which we see the world has been cleaned.

With muscle testing, the tester needs to be in the higher altitudes for the results to be valid. If someone is in fear or anger, the muscle testing will be "tainted" by the level of the tester.

Chapter 10
Archetypes
Muscle Testing Exercise

An archetype is a universal set of behaviors that would describe a pattern or role or label. Mother, author, hermit, nurse, teacher, leader, and organizer are all archetypes. We know an author writes, a teacher teaches, and an organizer organizes.

We each have a number of different archetypes. Our archetypes play valuable roles in our lives, work, and relationships. They influence everything we do, think, and feel. Our archetypes help us to learn about our spirituality, finances, and values. They are expressions of the inner self. Archetypes tap into the emotions of our inner world and give life a sense of personal meaning.

Archetypes can be career-orientated such as a businessman, nurse, or teacher. Some might describe personal traits such diva, hermit, or knight. Some might be hobbies such as music, photography, or sports. Others might be roles we play in our lives like father, friend, or sage.

Archetypes are diverse and many. We each have our own archetypes that are unique to us. The archetype influences how we interpret our world. The dreamer archetype will most certainly interact with the world differently than the intellectual.

The hermit will respond differently than the companion archetype. The innovator sees the future whereas the bureaucrat archetype might be stuck in the past. The storyteller might view life as a narrative whereas the rebel is in the middle of the narrative.

Archetypes are neutral by nature: neither good nor bad, favorable or unfavorable. Each archetype has a "light" side and a "dark" side. The child, for example, could be the joyous, happy child or the kid from hell. The mother archetype: Could be the loving mom that nurture her child or the "helicopter" mom that "hovers," controls, and bubble wraps their child every time they step outside the door.

We have the same archetypes throughout our lives. Archetypes come "online" at different times in our lives. For example:

* For the first twenty years of my life, my athlete archetype was central in my life. I started ballet when I was three years old. When I was seven, I told my mom I wanted to join the swim team. I started teaching swimming when I was twelve years old. Both my BS and MA degrees are in physical education.

* In my twenties and thirties, I started a company that manufactured greeting cards and stationery. My business archetype was most definitely central at that time.

* In my forties, fifties and sixties, my life coach, organizer, and author archetypes were central. Learning EFT Tapping, creating tapping statements, then organizing the statements and writing a story for the statements has been central.

Carolyn Myss teaches that we all have 12 primary Archetypes, four that are Universal (child, victim, saboteur, and prostitute) and eight that are uniquely our own.

The four Universal archetypes are important
to everyone's growth. They can become
our greatest teachers.

* Who better to point out when we are playing victim than the victim?

* Who better to tell us how to overcome our tendencies to sabotage our success than the saboteur?

* And the prostitute? They teach us where we sell out, compromise our integrity, morals, talents, ideals, or other expressions of our being for financial gain. The unhappy wife that prefers to stay in a loveless marriage rather than to be on her own, financially responsible for herself. The employee that becomes a workaholic to satisfy a tryant of a boss. These would be the prostitute archetype.

THESE FOUR UNIVERSAL ARCHETYPES CAN BECOME
OUR MOST TRUSTED PARTNERS AND TEACHERS.

One of my clients, Joyce, had a sense that one of her siblings, the one that was taking care of their aging parents, was doing something unethical. She felt she was being victimized by her brother, but not knowing how. She decided to have her parents' financial accounts audited without the brother's knowledge. She discovered the brother was secretly withdrawing funds from their parents' account for his own personal use.

She wasn't victimizing herself. She did feel it was her victim archetype that caused the funny feeling in her stomach every time she talked to the sibling that alerted her to something wasn't quite right.

The list of archetypes is on the next page. The page following the list of archetypes will describe varies way of determining your primary archetypes.

List of Archetypes

Actor
Actress
Administrator
Adventurer
Advocate
Alchemist
Ambassador
Analyst
Apprentice
Architect
Archaeologist
Artist
Athlete
Author
Banker
Bookkeeper
Builder
Business
Caregiver
Chef
Child (Universal)
Clown
Coach
Comedian
Communicator
Companion
Connoisseur
Counselor
Craftsman
Creator
Critic
Dancer
Daredevil
Defender
Designer
Detective
Dilettante
Diplomat
Director

Diva
Doctor
Don Juan
Drama
Dreamer
Drifter
Economist
Editor
Educator
Emperor
Empress
Engineer
Entrepreneur
Eccentric
Evangelist
Examiner
Explorer
Farmer
Father
Flirt
Friend
Gambler
Gardener
Gossip
Guide
Healer
Hermit
Hero
Heroine
Historian
Humanitarian
Innovator
Instructor
Intellectual
Inventor
Investigator
Jester
Journalist
Judge

Justice
King
Knight
Leader
Liberator
Lifeguard
Lover
Manager
Mathematician
Mediator
Medicine
Mentor
Military
Minister
Monk
Mother
Musician
Mystic
Networker
Nun
Nurse
Nurturer
Orator
Organizer
Peacemaker
Performer
Planner
Phoenix
Photographer
Pilot
Pioneer
Poet
Police
Politician
Preacher
Priest
Priestess
Prince
Princess

Professor
Prostitute Universal)
Protector
Publisher
Queen
Rebel
Reporter
Rescuer
Revolutionary
Robin Hood
Romantic
Saboteur (Universal)
Sage
Scholar
Scientist
Secretary
Seeker
Seer
Servant
Shaman
Sidekick
Singer
Slave
Solider
Spy
Storyteller
Student
Teacher
Theologian
Therapist
Thinker
Traveler
Victim (Universal)
Visionary
Wanderer
Warrior
Wizard
Workaholic
Writer

How Do We Determine Our Archetypes

Through self-reflection and/or muscle testing:

1) If we look back at our lives, we might find patterns. Seventy years ago, it was not okay for little girls to be athletic. I didn't care. I liked being physical as a dancer, swimmer, and in any sport I could play or participate in. The athlete has been a primary archetype for me since the day I was born.

For you, it might have been the rebel, artist, knight, explorer, or the builder.

2) An archetype could be aligned with our career such as actor, teacher, detective, scientist, minister, or farmer.

3) An archetype might be an important characteristic that defines who we are, separate from our profession, such as intellectual, lover, poet, or theologian.

4) An archetype could be something we are drawn to, yet it might not be a part of our lives at this time; however, we might want to pursue and learn more about. These are archetypes such as visionary, writer, healer, inventor, therapist, or scholar.

In looking at the list, you might notice some are very similar. For example, the teacher, guide, educator, mentor, or instructor. Which could it be for you? Whichever you resonate with the most. Each of us may have a different definition for the same word.

Going though the list, you might find 20 or 30 or 40 potential archetypes. Indicate them in some way and then determine if some of them go together.

For instance:

* Wanderer and traveler might be combined. To determine which is primary, ask which is most important. Is traveling more important than wandering or wandering is the way in which you enjoy traveling?

* Editor, writer, author, storyteller. Which is most important? Does the storyteller become an author and, thus storytelling is more important? Or does the author want to include stories in their writing to illustrate a narrative?

* Innovator, entrepreneur, and business. Which is primary? The innovator who has a wonderful idea? The entrepreneur that enjoys being their own boss and thus, decides to take an innovative idea to the market place?

Caroline Myss teaches that each of us has eight primary archetypes that are unique to us. Then each of us has an additional four that are universal...Child, Prostitute, Saboteur, and Victim.

Which eight archetypes are unique to you?
1.

2.

3.

4.

5.

6.

7.

8.

Now that you have determined the eight archetypes that are unique to you, the next chapter will teach you how to use these archetypes to find what may fulfill you.

Chapter 11
Finding Our Fulfillment

The inside of our rut and comfort zone, most likely, is not fulfilling. One reason to venture outside our comfort zone is to find fulfillment. Have you thought of what might be fulfilling for you? Have you thought about what your life might be missing? Do you have a reason to leave your comfort zone?

What if finding fulfillment could be as simple as a "formula?"

Determining what would be fulfilling might be that easy. The hard part might actually be stepping out of our comfort zone.

FOUR STEPS TO FINDING YOUR FULFILLMENT

1. Identify the archetype.
2. Identify the what.
3. Identify the why.
4. Follow through on what the archetype needs to do.

You have determined your archetypes. Here is a list of potential "Whats" and "Whys"

To accomplish	To evolve	To love
To achieve	To focus	To mastery
To take action	To give back	To be brave
To connect	To grow	To be bold
To endure	To heal	To be cheerful
To excel	To lead	To be competent
To explore	To learn	To be confident

To be creative	To be healthy	To be persistent
To be courageous	To be imaginative	To be playful
To be curious	To be independent	To be proficient
To be daring	To be inspirational	To be reliable
To be decisive	To be inventive	To be resilient
To be dependable	To be joyful	To be resourceful
To be dynamic	To be kind	To be responsible
To be easygoing	To be mindful	To be self-reliant
To be effective	To be nurturing	To be serene
To be empathetic	To be open-minded	To be tranquil
To be energetic	To be open	To be truthful
To be enlightened	To be organized	To be unique
To be enthusiastic	To be passionate	To be wise

FULFILLMENT FORMULA

The "formula" could look something like this:

As an actor, I find fulfillment by playing roles that allow me to express my creativity.

As a ____[who]____, I find fulfillment by _____[what] _____ to _____[why]_____.

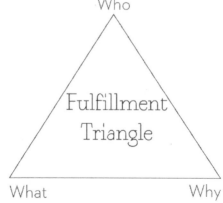

Determining What Would Be Fulfilling

To feel fulfilled, we must discover the who, what, and why. The "who" is the archetype, the "what" is what they need to do, and the "why" is why they need to do what they need to do. Discovering the "what" and "why" is equally as important as the "who."

When an archetype comes "online" and we either are unaware or don't allow the archetype a role in our lives, we can feel somewhat out of synch with ourselves, like something is missing. An archetype not being able to fulfill their 'what' and their 'why' could result in us not feeling fulfilled.

Examples of an archetype, their what, and their why:

* An actor might find fulfillment by playing roles that allow them to express their creativity.
  Who – an actor
  What – playing roles
  Why – to express their creativity

* A banker might find fulfillment by helping others not to be overwhelmed with the process of buying a home.
  Who – a banker
  What – helping others
  Why – so the client is not overwhelmed

* A businesswoman might find fulfillment by creating her own income to be able to be her own boss and work the hours that allow her to raise a family.
  Who – a businesswoman
  What – creating her own income
  Why – to be her own boss and be able to create her own work hours

* An athlete might find fulfillment by focusing on their health to be able to improve the quality of their life.

      Who – the athlete

      What – focusing on their health

      Why – to improve the quality of their life

* A teacher might find fulfillment by teaching children the lessons of life to better prepare them to navigate the real world.

      Who – a teacher

      What – teaching children the lessons of life

      Why – To better prepare them to navigate the real world

IT'S NOT JUST DISCOVERING THE "WHO"; IT IS EQUALLY AS IMPORTANT TO DISCOVER THEIR "WHAT" AND THEIR "WHY".

New Product Launching Fall 2023

Tessa created a new series call *Awaken, Emerge, Become* to provide a guide for a seeker to find their own insights and ah-ha wisdom. The series includes a book, card deck, journal, and Workbook and work in tandem with each other.

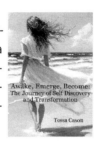

The book, *Awaken, Emerge, Become: The Journey of Self-Reflection and Transformation* is a step-by-step guide from self discovery to transformation. It includes many of the tools, techniques, and methods she learned from some remarkable teachers.

The sixty card deck, *Awaken, Emerge, Become: Card Deck of Exploration* is a fun tool to aid in finding answers, discover new insights, and might provide new awarenesses for the inquisitive.

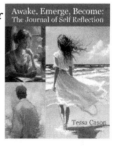

Awaken, Emerge, Become: The Journal of Self-reflection is a series of questions to help a seeker discern their truths. The intent of the journal is to assist you in finding your ah-ha wisdom, answers to the challenges you currently are facing, and possible paths to healing physically, mentally, emotionally, and spiritually.

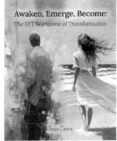

Awaken, Emerge, Become: The EFT Workbook for Transformation is a step-by-step guide to becoming the highest potential of ourselves.

Books by Tessa Cason

80 EFT TAPPING STATEMENTS FOR:
Abandonment
Abundance, Wealth, Money
Addictions
Adult Children of Alcoholics
Anger and Frustration
Anxiety and Worry
Change
"Less Than" and Anxiety
Manifesting a Romantic Relationship
Relationship with Self
Self Esteem
Social Anxiety
Weight and Emotional Eating

100 EFT Tapping Statements for Accepting Our Uniqueness
and Being Different
100 EFT Tapping Statements for Being Extraordinary!
100 EFT Tapping Statements for Fear of Computers
100 EFT Tapping Statements for Feeling Deserving
100 EFT Tapping Statements for Feeling Fulfilled
200 EFT Tapping Statements for Conflict
200 EFT Tapping Statements for Healing a Broken Heart
200 EFT Tapping Statements for Knowing God
200 EFT Tapping Statements for Positive Thinking vs
Positive Avoidance
200 EFT Tapping Statements for Procrastination
200 EFT Tapping Statements for PTSD
200 EFT Tapping Statements for Sex

200 EFT Tapping Statements for Wealth
240 EFT Tapping Statements for Fear
300 EFT Tapping Statements for Healing the Self
300 EFT Tapping Statements for Dealing with Obnoxious People
300 EFT Tapping Statements for Intuition
300 EFT Tapping Statements for Self-defeating Behaviors,
Victim, Self-pity
340 EFT Tapping Statements for Healing From the Loss
of a Loved One
400 EFT Tapping Statements for Being a Champion
400 EFT Tapping Statements for Being Empowered
and Successful
400 EFT Tapping Statements for Dealing with Emotions
400 EFT Tapping Statements for Dreams to Reality
400 EFT Tapping Statements for My Thyroid Story
500 EFT Tapping Statements for Moving Out of Survival
700 EFT Tapping Statements for Weight, Emotional Eating,
and Food Cravings
All Things EFT Tapping Manual
Emotional Significance of Human Body Parts
Muscle Testing – Obstacles and Helpful Hints

EFT TAPPING STATEMENTS FOR:
A Broken Heart, Abandonment, Anger, Depression,
Grief, Emotional Healing
Anxiety, Fear, Anger, Self Pity, Change
Champion, Success, Personal Power, Self Confidence,
Leader/Role Model
Prosperity, Survival, Courage, Personal Power, Success
PTSD, Disempowered, Survival, Fear, Anger
Weight & Food Cravings, Anger, Grief, Not Good Enough,
Failure

Printed in Great Britain
by Amazon

29426373R00051